Teaching Kids About Bullying

How To Fight Bullying By Teaching Kids Emotional Skills And Social Skills

Frank Dixon

Table of Contents

Introduction

"But I don't want to go to school today. My stomach hurts…"

This seems to be the common plight of every fourth or sixth-grader, and as parents, we often disregard it as blatant excuses to skip school. But how many of us have stopped to wonder why our child has started to make excuses to go to school? Why does he drag his feet when you repeatedly tell him to get dressed fast? Statistics from the National Bullying Prevention Centre show that children, boys, in particular, are victims of bullying and physical assault in schools. It is estimated that each year some 160,000 kids refuse to go to school because they are bullied, harassed, called names, insulted, or made fun of, as per National Centre for Education Statistics and Bureau of Justice. Boys have it harder when it comes to bullying and are more likely to become a victim of verbal and physical harassments than girls. Girls engage in relational bullying where they try to act superior to one another in terms of looks and appearance.

We assume that it is something that would never happen to our child. Why would anyone want to hurt a sweet boy or be mean to a sweet girl? Besides, they look well. They may look well and composed on the outside, but inside, they are battling with themselves every single day.

Bullying is a common disease - a chronic disease that leaves its victims weak, suppressed, and hollow. About 20% of all school-going kids are bullied, and these are just the statistics that are reported nationwide. The percentage would be higher if all bullied students remain silent or think that it is their fault. Students in their teen years report being bullied the most, but it can start a lot younger. Several surveys (Youth Risk Behavior Surveillance System (YRBSS), 2020) that tried to pin the image on a bully reveal that a bully can influence others' perception about their victim (56%), they have more social influence (50%), are stronger physically (40%), and have more money to get away with it (31%).

Most of the bullying occurs in hallways, classrooms, and cafeteria or on school grounds. Locker rooms and bathrooms are also notorious for easy prey.

The reason to share these statistics here today is to help you notice the severity of the crime that takes place and how we can put an end to it. As parents and educators, it is our job to intervene at the right time before it escalates. Additionally, we have the responsibility to teach our kids the right social and emotional skills to combat acts of bullying at school, on the bus, and anywhere else in a stringent manner and not let bullies get away with their harassing and teasing.

Teaching them strong emotional and social skills will help them become assertive and independent. It will help them stand up for those who can't stand up for themselves and report it to the authorities before it gets worse.

Several statistics suggest that revenge due to bullying is the primary motivator behind school shootings in the US. 75% of school shootings are linked to bullying and harassment.

Teachers have also been reported to have turned down students when they complain of being bullied or have witnessed someone getting bullied. They downplay and pretend that it isn't as serious, but some reports suggest that bullying can go on for approximately six months or longer. This can take away a child's mental peace and harm their mental health, self-esteem, and confidence. Research supports the idea that persistent bullying can lead to feelings of isolation, exclusion, and despair, which can turn to depression and anxiety.

As a parent, you wouldn't wish it on your child or any other. Our children are the most precious little people to us. We have kept them safe from all sorts of harm when they couldn't protect themselves. So why stop now? Now that they are growing up and handling their affairs on their own, don't you think they need our guidance more than ever? Learn to identify the warning signs whether your child is being bullied or worse is one because research suggests that 64% of those who are bullied never report it.

In this next guide, we look at what bullying is, how to classify it, its various forms and how we can teach our kids to be emotionally and socially stable to put an end to it. Sometimes, all it takes is someone to clap back or intervene to stop a bully in action. Let your children be strong enough to defend themselves and brave enough to intervene and put an end to bullying.

Chapter 1:

Bullying: Humiliating, Disrespecting, and Harming Others for Personal Pleasure

Bullying is defined as a power imbalance between two or more opponents where the privileged one gets to exert power both mentally and physically onto the weaker one. Most of the time, bullying begins with verbal abuse and can sometimes escalate to being physical. Bullying in schools and colleges is a common incidence and often the one most unreported. It can take the form of verbally abusing others by calling them names, using slurs, cruel teasing, or discriminating a kid out for being of a different race, religion, or sexual orientation. Bullying isn't always confrontational. It can be via various channels like phone via text messaging or through social media platforms.

When we think of bullying, we look at it from three different components. The first is intention. Intention refers to the act of being deliberately hurtful or aggressive towards someone. No one likes to admit that they are rude or being mean to another on purpose; however, that has been their intent from the get-go. It can be unintentional where the goal isn't to cause harm or hurt to someone but to joke a bit to make others laugh. But it must never be at the expense of someone that might take offense.

The second is a power grab. The bully must have power over the victim to intimidate them. Without power, a bully isn't considered a bully. He may be an influencer of sorts that targets weaker opponents, but he can't be called a bully. This power grab becomes stronger as the bully gains more confidence and momentum. There comes a time when bullies start to get off with the pleasure that comes from putting others down. They get addicted to the attention and fame that they receive. They admire the sight when others refrain from getting in their way and fear them.

The final component is repeated assault action. Repeated actions suggest an ongoing pattern of bad behavior. The bully repeatedly says or does mean and negative things to someone either face-to-face or from behind a screen. The goal is to purposely exclude the victim from a group or activity or make a laughing stock of them.

Bullying creates a negative culture of fear among tweens and teenagers. It impacts the lives of all those that are involved in it, yes, even the bully and the bystander. It distorts the mental peace and health of the victim, makes the bystander question their values and self-esteem, and causes the bully to struggle with anger and control issues later in life. Being bullied can take a physical, emotional, and mental toll on a person's well-being. It can result in poor grades and loss of confidence. It can leave the victim feeling isolated and left out. Someone who is being bullied might also start to think negatively about themselves and have vengeful and suicidal thoughts.

It all starts with a little bit of joking and teasing and later turns into hazing and harassment. As a parent, you might think all these terms mean the same thing, but there are slight differences that determine the level of bullying. Each term also has different implications for its victims. For example, kids who are teased occasionally might forget about it later in life and learn to brush it off. However, someone that has been harassed or violated in some way might never get over it and forever live with the fear of it happening again.

In this first chapter, we are going to explore these differences to develop a better understanding of what your child is experiencing. This will also help you help them out in a compassionate and understanding manner.

Bullying and Teasing

Teasing isn't always bad. Good-natured teasing can be an excellent way to communicate with one another. It is rather common among a group of friends and often light-hearted. Think of it as a social exchange. Some kids get offended by it in the meantime, but it doesn't cause any long-term damage to their self-esteem. They can also be the reason for a strong bond formation as laughter and joy are known to bring people together. For example, while walking in the hallway, a kid trips over, and the other friend says something like, Hey, nice one. They both can laugh it off and still be friends.

Teasing, if done in the right spirit, can be positive. Teachers can tease their children by assigning them names based on their personalities, and everyone might love them more. Children can tease one another about clothes, movie or song tastes, or behavior. It can also be constructive in many ways.

Then, good-natured teasing can be done to influence one another to improve behavior. For example, if one kid at school has a crush on a girl, a friend might comment something like, "Hey, you are still looking at her, just go over and say hi." This is both constructive feedback and improvement in one's behavior.

Teasing can be mean too. It can communicate the negative. A child may use it as a means to become the top dog among their peers. For instance, a girl might frequently tease another friend about her increasing weight, the number of pimples on her face, or her taste in boys. Some might also use it to encourage bad behavior, like a boy calling his friend a wimp for not trying a cigarette.

Additionally, the statements or things said may not be as playful as initially thought and end up making the other feel worthless or ashamed. For example, talking bad about someone's skin color or sexual orientation may not always be the right way to get a laugh. It can lead to hurt feelings.

Teasing usually has an intention and purpose. It can involve verbal abuse and become bullying, especially when it is done to people that aren't good friends. Then, the goal changes from just joking to embarrassing someone. Bullying often starts as casual teasing. When a bully notices the kind of attention and laughter it gets them; they start to repeat that behavior and pick on those that seem defenseless. Teasing becomes bullying when:

- The nature of the content turns from affectionate to hostile.
- The teasing occurs frequently.
- There is a power imbalance.
- The teaser means to hurt or upsets the one being teased.
- The teased is upset by the interaction even though they might not show it.

Bullying and Harassment

Bullying and harassment may look the same to many; however, they differ from one another based on the intensity of the crime. The difference lies in the presence of laws and protection for students and children that are harassed. When we talk about bullying, we talk about an act or behavior that is intended to harm or hurt another, cause them humiliation, and attack them personally. There is usually an imbalance of power where the bully feels more in control of their victim and uses that power to influence others. It could be social standing, wealth, or the number of people on their side.

When we talk of harassment, we talk about unwanted and hurtful actions that include unwelcome verbal abuse, threats, assaults, or misconduct of other similar sorts. The assault may also come in the form of sharing graphic content, such as threatening a student to leak a tape of them doing drugs or share revealing pictures online unless they do something in return. Harassment can be based on a student's race, religion, age, sex, color, disability, or national origin. For example, demeaning someone for their disability is both harassment and bullying.

Bullying and Hazing

Hazing is another big issue in high schools and colleges. Surveys conclude that more than 50% of college students who are part of a team, club, or other organization have experienced being hazed at some point. 47% of high schoolers have experienced hazing before even entering college. The most common form of hazing students experience includes humiliation, sleep deprivation, sexual acts, isolation, and binge drinking. The difference between bullying and hazing is subtle but present. The same power dynamics are involved in hazing as well as bullying. There is intimidation involved too. However, the distinctive feature remains that in hazing, a hazer makes someone commit crimes that can be harmful to them. In bullying, one singles out a victim and tries to exclude them from the group. In hazing, if someone wishes to earn their way into the group, they have to do dangerous stuff or mock themselves first. Bullies usually work alone or can have a few other people. Hazing is done mainly by an entire group or team. Take sororities or frat houses as an example. If you want to join, you have to have a particular skill or talent or do something to earn a place. You don't just get included otherwise.

Hazing can take several forms. It can include:

- Yelling or swearing insults at the victim

- Depriving the victim of necessities like food or a bed to sleep on
- Restricting personal hygiene
- Insisting the victim get involved in sexual acts
- Beating, restraining, gagging, or whipping victims
- Forcing victims to eat or drink something vile
- Forcing binge eating or drinking
- Branding the victim in some way

Chapter 2:

Is My Child Being Bullied?

Although the signs aren't always there, and teenagers tend to hide the fact that they are bullied at school or online, it is still vital as a parent to know what's going on in the life of your child. Bullying is something not everyone is capable of handling alone. They need guidance, compassion, and assertiveness to deal with what's happening to them and how they can put an end to it. However, before we get to the preventive part, the following three chapters are going to involve profiling a victim, a bully, and a bystander. Since these three play a crucial role, we must know what they look like and how to decipher any warning signs early on.

Profiling: The Victim

Bullying can take many forms. The victims of bullying are affected the most as they are the central target of mocking, teasing, and harassment. Bullies often prey on those that appear defenseless, which means that the victim is someone that has a weak sense of confidence and worth. But this doesn't characterize them. A victim can be a chubby rich kid with a disability mocked by a shorter and petite kid from a middle-class background. So how can you profile a victim? How can you know if your child is a victim of bullying or not if there is nothing prominent?

Not every victim might look or act like it, but some distinct characteristics are most commonly reported among those bullied.

Kids that are bullied don't have a lot of friends. They are often loners and, therefore, an easy target. They appear weaker than those that are in a group or are well-known by their classmates and teachers. When you are in a group, you always have their support. You aren't easy to pick on. As one of the primary components of bullying is the power grab, a lack of social support from peers and teachers allows the bully to appear more powerful than the one they intend to bully.

Bully victims are often those with special needs or learning disabilities. For instance, autistic kids are more prone to bullying than other kids (Rowley et al., 2012).

Tweens and teenagers that appear submissive, anxious, or passive are more likely to be bullied than those that don't exhibit these traits, as per research (Hong et al., 2011). Bullied kids are more insecure and prone to crying when jilted a little. This makes it more fun for the bully to take on them.

A lack of assertiveness, as stated above, can also be one of the reasons that make someone a target for bullying.

Kids who suffer from mental health issues like depression or stress are also more likely to become prey (Gini & Pozzoli, 2013). These problems are only worsened by the ongoing bullying.

Victims of bullying are often not accepted by other kids. Bystanders that witness bullying in action don't want to be associated with the victim in any way because it makes them a target too. Victims experience peer rejection and are on their own in social events, one of the many reasons they prefer to stay at home than attend a social affair at school.

Children perceived as different are also more likely to be bullied. This includes children that resonate with different sexual orientations. For example, many boys have to suppress their inner feelings and go on dates with girls because they fear their friends will make fun of them if they come out.

Children that stand out from the crowd for any apparent reasons can become an easy target.

- They might be from a different race, culture, or religion.
- They may be from the LGBTQ community.
- They may have a special talent or are nerdy.
- They have a physical or mental disorder.

Some studies suggest that children, both boys, and girls that are overweight or larger, are prone to becoming victims of bullying. They may be bigger, but they are rather conscious about the way they look. Children that reach puberty earlier than their peers or years after them are also susceptible to bullying.

Warning Signs My Child is a Victim of Bullying

Now that you have a better picture of a victim of bullying or at least have an idea of whether your child is a target or not, below are some risk signs that confirm your doubts. If your child is being bullied, they will:

- Come home with clothes that are torn
- Have bruises or injuries on their hands, face, or upper body
- Never bring their classmates to their home for group study
- Not have a special friend they can confide in
- Show reluctance to go to school
- Not gets invited to school parties
- Experience restlessness and suffer from sleep deprivation
- Lose interest in academics and hobbies they enjoyed before
- Choose illogical routes to go to school
- Steal money from you or your spouse

If you notice any of these signs, especially if your child comes home with unexplained injuries or has bruises on their chest or side of the waist, it is best to intervene and question. However, there is a way to go about it. Keep in mind that there is a reason why your child didn't confide in you in the first place. They could have easily come to you and told you that they were being harassed. The reason they didn't is that they thought they could handle it themselves. They still do! Or they don't want to worry you unconditionally because they believe that you are already stressed or too busy to focus on them. They might also think that talking to you will only make things worse for them at school because the administration will get involved, and they will have to testify against the bully.

However, if it is chipping away their mental health, affecting their studies, and causing them distress, adults must arbitrate. In chapter 6, we shall discuss the best way to initiate a healthy and compassionate conversation with your child and help them stand up to their bully or find other means to put the bullying at bay.

Chapter 3:

Or Worse... A Bully?

A bully is made when a kid or adult decides they need to have more control over someone. The aggression that a bully builds up interferes with the empathy in them. Without this empathy, they can't refrain from bullying others. We define this aggression in two forms: proactive and reactive.

Proactive aggressors are organized, driven by a desire to control, and emotionally detached.

Proactive aggression is described as being organized, emotionally detached, and driven by the desire for a reward. Reactive aggression is linked with intense emotion, an impulsive nature, and a response to a perceived threat. Unlike those who had been victims of bullying themselves, bullies who are proactive have high self-esteem and are social climbers. Bullies, in general, have a low tolerance for anger, frustration and have trouble empathizing. They are more likely to battle mental health issues that make them act irrationally, angrily, and at times, crazy. Non-victimized bullies are bi-strategic controllers. They use both prosocial actions and negative actions like coercing, intimidation and assault to engage in harmful behavior towards others.

Bullies that were victims themselves of the heinous crime are more aggressive in general than those who have never been bullied. These bullies are less popular, come from families of low socioeconomic standing, and have been abused, bullied, or neglected by their siblings or parents.

In this chapter, we explore the makings of a bully and how parents determine if their child is a bully or becoming one. Later, we briefly look at the different types of bullies to further understand the nature of a bully and what causes them to become one.

The Makings of a Bully

To paint a typical picture of a bully, imagine someone that is:

- Physically aggressive
- Verbally abusive
- Confident
- Positive views over violence
- Low tolerance for frustration
- Impulsive
- Strong need to dominate
- Physically stronger
- Little empathy
- Popular

- Is skilled to get themselves out of tricky situations
- Blames the victim for being weak, different, or poor
- Has been exposed to violence or bullying at an early age
- Has adults in their lives that model violence
- Lack of respect for others

These are some qualities that make a bully stand out. Most of these are easily distinguishable.

Warning Signs My Child is a Bully

Kids that were bullied before can become the same thing they hated. Bullying others becomes an outlet for such kids to vent out pent-up anger and frustration. When they see someone else suffering or being hurt, it makes them feel empowered and in control – the two things they lacked when they were bullied. As most of the bullying starts at home for them, many parents remain unaware that their child has become one. To them, arguing with adults, not listening to them, disregarding their opinions, acting crazy are all normal symptoms of growing up. Some parents are inattentive or abusive, which makes the child mentally unstable, leading to becoming a bully. When they get abused at home, scolded, or hit, they feel powerless. Bullying kids weaker than them restores that sense of power and control.

However, if it has come to your notice that your child has become a bully or if you are unsure about their behavior, below are some signs to confirm your doubts and take immediate action.

The things you should look for in your child if they are a bully include:

- Teasing everyone in a nasty manner, often those who are defenseless and weak
- Appearing stronger physically and enjoy watching violence-based shows on TV
- Wanting to dominate and use threats to control others
- Being impulsive and easily-angered
- Being aggressive towards adults
- Being unsympathetic towards others and hardened
- Thinking no one is better than themselves
- Engaging in negative acts such as cheating, lying, or disrespecting others
- Being poor in studies and have lower than average grades

Types of Bullies

Bullies have different goals, styles, personalities, and behaviors. Some resort to just verbal abuse when trying to overpower their victims, while some go beyond that. Some work solo while others rely on their friends to help them. Every bully's motivation to bully and method is different. It is hard to put them neatly into just one category. For example, some bullies are both verbally and physically abusive. In this section, we discuss some basic categories that you should know of so that you are both on the same page when you get down to have a conversation with your child about it. The more you know, the better strategies you can advise and implement to help your child stand up against a bully or stop from becoming one.

Bully-Victims

These are those that rise after being bullied. They prey on those that are weaker than them in appearance. They were once the same, and as stated before, their ultimate goal is to regain a sense of control and power.

This is a very common type of bully. A large number of boys who had been bullied by their peers fall under this category. They bully because they want to retaliate against the pain they suffered. These bullies come from households where bullying goes unattended. Usually, the parents are least concerned, and the siblings are scary and abusive. Whenever, in the beginning, they went up to their parents to complain about an incident of bullying, they were told to 'man up' and take matters into their own hands. So they did.

This form of behavior is, therefore, learned. The majority of such bullies are loners and at the bottom of the social ladder. This only adds to their sense of powerlessness. It makes them feel angry and frustrated. They want to be seen, be feared the same way they fear a sibling or a parent, and use hostile methods to tease their victims.

Popular Bullies

These bullies come packed with big egos. They are fearless, condescending, and confident of themselves. They are on top of the social ladder in school and have a following. Imagine big jocks, a captain of the basketball team, and someone who thinks everyone owes them respect and love. They feel like they rule the world. Their sense of entitlement stems from their popularity, size, upbringing, or socioeconomic status.

Popular bullies thrive on the control and physical power that they have over their victims. They don't pick hallway corners or locker rooms to bully their victim. They do it in the open, where everyone can see them being in control. Since they have a huge following and everyone is afraid of them, students don't tell on them. They aren't afraid of being called out for bullying either. If anything, they like to boast about it.

The methods they use often involve:

- Pushing the victim.
- Stalking them.
- Taking their lunch.
- Tearing their notebooks.
- Pinning them against the lockers.

Girls aren't far behind either. They resort to the same behaviors, but their interest is more towards relational aggression. They would rather just spread lies, manipulate their victim, or start rumors to exclude others than push, kick, or pin them against a locker.

Popular bullies are star kids, and they thrive on the attention and power they gain from bullying. The #1 reason their peers don't tell on them is that they would rather be accepted by them than be bullied.

Indifferent Bullies

As the name suggests, these bullies are indifferent toward any pain they cause. They lack empathy. They are unable to feel the harm they cause. They act cold, emotionally detached, and don't let remorse get to them. They enjoy being able to cause pain. These types of bullies are the most dangerous but, thankfully, rare.

Indifferent bullies recharge themselves when they see another person's suffering. There isn't always a motivation behind the hatred they feel towards someone. They don't fear disciplinary action against them. These bullies have severe mental health issues and psychological problems. They often require therapy and are seen by a professional. Using traditional methods like talking or counseling doesn't help them change or become a better person. They need in-depth treatment to get over the privileged mindset they have and view others as humans. What makes them so vicious is still debatable; however, some research into them reveals that the reason they feel no empathy is because they have been exposed to violence at an early age and have built a wall around themselves to prevent anyone from hurting them anymore. They will purposely hurt innocent animals for fun and expect others to celebrate them.

Relational Bullies

Relational bullies like to be in control. If you want to picture a relational bully, imagine someone popular with a big following and a central member of a large group that decides who is accepted at school and who isn't. Relational bullies use methods like isolation, banishment, and exclusion. They don't resort to physical means of bullying. Their words are enough to cause emotional pain. They take away a victim's power. Since they are popular in school, people fear them. Bystanders don't want to be the ones to rat on them because they fear they will be bullied in return. Popular girls make up most of this category.

Relational bullies also use labels, name-calling, spreading rumors, and lies about their victim. Often the motive behind is jealousy. If they fear that someone might become more popular, loved, or socially acceptable than them, they try to exclude them. They can't do without their popularity and therefore will do whatever it takes to maintain it. Relational bullies want the whole world to revolve around, and anyone that tries to challenge that or take away the spotlight becomes a target.

Group Bullies

Bullies, in this category, work as a team and have a pack mentality. They work together to bring someone down. Usually, there is a leader that leads the pack, and the remaining members act as collaborators. For example, if the leader is the one punching the victim, the remaining friends will be the ones restricting the kid in place while others watch out for an adult. You will be surprised how differently they will act when not around their friends. Even when alone with the victim, they act differently. Group bullies are commonly cliques that imitate the actions and behaviors of their leader. They are merely followers of a superior bully.

This is a dangerous type of bullying as things can escalate real fast, especially when the victim isn't backing down or trying to defend themselves. This also suggests that group bullies fear being caught and aren't methodological. When in the group, they feel less responsible for the outcomes because they know that their friends will be at their side.

Serial Bullies

Finally, we have a serial bully that is yet another popular type of bully. Serial bullies are controlled, systematic, and calculated in their methods. They will appear sweet, charismatic, and often charming towards the teachers and principal. They act as if they are the most responsible of students and the most caring. But to their peers and students younger than them, they are known to inflict pain. They rarely resort to physical bullying as they know they can rely on just verbal slurs. Kids are afraid of them because of the immense power they hold. Serial bullies know that even if someone were to rat them out to a teacher, the teacher wouldn't believe the victim.

Serial bullies have fake friends, are skilled manipulators, and liars. Their sugary persona is a smart way to manipulate others to their liking. They can twist the facts and make themselves come out as the victim in a given situation. This makes getting out of trouble easy.

Chapter 4:

Bystanders – The Supporting Cast in the Drama

This brings us to our final players in the act – perhaps the only cast that can turn the tables around and surprise everyone with their classic improvisation and receive applause and praise from the audiences – the bystanders.

If bystanders intervene at the right time and stop a bully from gaining power over a victim, things wouldn't get out of hand. Simply put, a bystander can be anyone that witnesses the bullying in person or via digital forms like text messages, social media, games, or websites. Research (Polanin et al., 2012) suggests that whenever an instance of bullying occurs, especially in schools or colleges, bystanders are present 80% of the time. A bystander holds the power to make a positive difference in a bullying situation by standing up in support of the victim and putting the bully in their place.

When a victim feels supported and defended, they can build the courage within to speak for themselves. When a bystander, particularly a senior or adult, intervenes, the incidence of bullying stops within ten seconds, 57% of the time.

However, not every bystander is aware of the power they hold or intervene at the right time. And why blame youngsters alone for their lack of confidence and willingness when we are no different. As adults, parents, and educators, how many times have we intervened and stopped a situation from becoming worse? How many times have we walked away telling ourselves that it isn't our business to engage? How many times have we looked the other way and told our children to do the same so that we can keep them safe?

Children are sponges. They soak up all that they see us doing. They imitate our actions and behaviors. They view us as their role models and are too naïve to know when we are in the wrong. Therefore, this makes for an important reminder. We must teach the right values so that our child doesn't fear speaking up for someone else in need. If they witness someone getting bullied, they must know the right thing to do and try to stop the bully from hurting the victim. If they can't do so, they must gather teachers or administration members to witness it for themselves and have the bully punished for their actions.

A bystander can play different roles in the event of bullying.

They can choose to be an outsider that only witnesses someone getting bullied but doesn't do anything about it. They can choose to be defenders and offer help by intervening or extending their support and friendship to the bullied, either privately or publicly. They can choose to be reinforcers that support the youth that bullies others or promotes such behavior. They may be the ones laughing or encouraging the bully to cause further harm to the bullied. Lastly, they can choose to be assistants to the bully and join in. For example, if the bully feels like punching a kid, they may physically restrain the victim or prevent them from getting away.

Why Bystanders Don't Step In

There are a number of reasons why bystanders don't wish to intervene, even when they know it is the right thing to do. Let's explore these reasons and try to understand what must go through the mind of a little child that witnessed bullying but hasn't got the guts to face the bully or defend the victim.

The #1 reason is fear of retaliation. Fear is also the reason why a victim doesn't report being bullied to their parents or educators. A bystander believes that if they intervene, it will make them the target too. This is especially true for someone who has been a victim of bullying previously. When they look at someone being bullied, they thank God that it isn't them.

Then, a bystander might also want to associate themselves with the bully because they view them as the stronger party. A bystander believes that if they join the kids that bully, it will prevent them from experiencing it. So they stay quiet because they want to be accepted. This is peer pressure at its best. However, if your child remains an innocent bystander when someone gets bullied, let them know that they shall have to be answerable one day.

A bystander is uncertain about what they must do. Confronting a bully isn't always the best means, especially if they are stronger, more powerful, and have a group of friends as their backup. A bystander knows that they have little hope of doing some actual prevention and, therefore, decide to ignore the bullying. If only they know better or are instructed on how they can help, many bullying incidents can be prevented.

They worry that if someone finds out that they were the ones that called upon the teachers to the scene, they will be labeled a snitch forever. Others will start to laugh at them for being a loser because they had to rely on others for help. It's like an unwritten rule among high school kids. No one wants to be labeled as a rat or a tattletale. Therefore, a bystander thinks so too and prefers to ignore or move on then do something about the bullying. Besides, being the one to call for help also makes them a target. They can't always hide from the bully, and if they know that it was the bystander that told on them, the bully and their friends are going to seek revenge.

Then, a bystander might also believe that their plea for help will be ignored, and nothing will be done about it after the teachers disperse the students. This lack of uncertainty is equally threatening. Despite official laws put in place against bullying, there are still some adults that would not believe a victim when they come to ask for help. They are told that they are being too sensitive, and it is merely some joking and teasing that a bully is doing. An adult might also try to encourage the bystander to take matters into their own hands. This makes the bystander apathetic about bullying. He knows it won't do anyone any good and move on.

A bystander might also not intervene because they think it is none of their business. After all, they aren't the ones getting verbally abused, kicked, or laughed at by others. Many parents teach their kids to do the same because they want to keep them safe and away from all sorts of violence. They tell their kids to keep to themselves and not try to act as a hero all the time. This is wrong on so many levels, and both parents and the child must be coached to act better and take responsibility when someone is being bullied.

A bystander might also believe that the victim deserves it. They might be new to the school or not know the reason behind why someone is being bullied. To stop themselves from intervening, they may tell themselves things like, "Maybe, the victim deserved it." To make themselves feel better about it, they assume that the victim is an annoying person and, therefore, deserving of their treatment. As adults, we know that this is rarely the case. A bully doesn't need a reason to attack someone. They do it for personal pleasure.

What Excuses Do Bystanders Give?

Apart from these reasons, there are several excuses a bystander might give when confronted and asked why they let a bullying situation escalate.

The most common excuse is not knowing what to do to make it stop. Even adults have a difficult time deciding whether they should deescalate a situation or not. They see someone become aggressive and can't decide if they should get involved or not. Their conscience tells them to intervene, but they don't know-how. Now imagine the same for a ten or fourteen-year-old child. So much goes into their minds. Schools have a crucial role to play here. They may have anti-bullying posters placed all over the school, talk about how bullying won't be acceptable on the school grounds, and talk about the many bullying-related tragedies. Yet fail to instruct kids how to effectively intervene when an adult is not available, or the bullying takes place elsewhere. Kids must be taught how to report, what they must say, and who to go to in case of having witnessed someone being bullied. They must be taught not to back away or ignore what's going on.

Another excuse common among bystanders is that the bully is their friend, and they aren't always bad. It isn't unusual to witness your friend bullying someone. For the other kids in the group, bullying is seen as a means to joke around and have fun. The group sees no harm in having a little fun and laughter. This is one of the many reasons a bully is never caught or afraid to take on the weaker kids. They have a strong support system, and they know that their friends won't rat them out. Friends of the bully are sometimes the first to have an issue with the victim, and then, they call in the bully to intervene and take things over. Some friends also start rumors about the victims and share them with their other friends. This further isolates the victim as no one wants to be associated with them.

Finally, a bystander might not intervene because they think since they don't know the victim personally nor are good friends with them. They think that it isn't their place to defend them. The fact that someone doesn't want to take responsibility and report the bullying suggests fear and ignorance. When bullying becomes too common, we begin to normalize that behavior. After some time, children become too used to seeing someone get bullied that it stops affecting them.

The Effects of Bullying on the Bystander

However, we must not undermine or ignore the impact an act of bullying has on the bystander. They may not be directly affected by the incident, but they deal with a lot of different emotions at the same time. One research study (Study shows bullying affects both bystanders and target, 2011) tried to study the effects of bullying on a bystander in more depth. They interviewed a group of 91 sixth-grader students to talk about whether they had seen someone being bullied or not and what their response was. They were questioned why they didn't tell anyone about it or if they did, whether something was done or not. They also sought more clarity on the emotions that a bystander went through when they witnessed someone getting physically assaulted in front of them.

Their answers revealed that they too suffered from negative consequences of the bullying and developed negative feelings of fear, guilt, stress, and reduced empathy. Those who witnessed bullying also demonstrated an increased heart rate and perspiration. Some of them also reported high levels of stress and trauma long after the event.

Most of the students reported fear as a common negative emotion followed by anxiety when they witnessed a bullying event. They live in fear that they will be the next target of the bully. They always look insecure and suffer from mental health problems that only escalate as they grow up. This loss of security prevents them from forming healthy friendships or trusting their friends.

Stress was the second most talked about emotion during the study. Students recalled having an increased heart rate as well as sweat on their forehead when they witnessed someone getting bullied. They also report poor concentration, a lack of focus, and a drop in their grades because they can't seem to forget or erase the memory from their heads. They also try to skip school as much as possible because they don't see it as a healthy environment.

A lot of students also report feeling guilty and ashamed for not defending the victim. Most of the students agreed that bullying was wrong and should be stopped. However, when questioned why they didn't do anything about it, they once again reported fear being the primary factor. So they feel guilty for and ashamed for letting the bully get away with the assault without paying a price. The students also talked about how this guilt and shame can manifest into poor decision-making and the consumption of drugs.

Reduced empathy was also another shocking effect. It was noticed that when the students that had witnessed multiple events of bullying talked about the events, there was a lack of empathy in their tones for the bullied. They had become so accustomed to the crime that they had lost all empathy for the person being bullied. It became an everyday nuisance to them that wasted everyone's time. They started to believe that the victim deserved it.

Chapter 5:

Different Shades of Bullies

Many people, who have been spared from being bullied, often wonder what it is and whether all bullying is the same or not. Surprisingly, we can classify the different types and forms of bullying based on their severity and instance. Some bullying is only verbal. It can sometimes escalate to physical assault. Some are done from behind a screen and don't involve face-to-face interaction. Some can be spotted easily, while some are more subtle and seldom. Some happen over a particular topic or interest, while other forms of bullying are more persistent and don't need a topic to begin. Some forms have moderate consequences, while other forms can be damaging to both physical and mental health. Some bullies rely on abusive slurs, while others are more competent at causing injury.

In all cases, a bully is the one with more power and command, whereas the victim is often viewed as defenseless and isolated.

In this next chapter, we are going to discuss six different types of bullying common in schools and colleges. We shall discuss their severity as well as their impact on the victim.

As a parent, this can serve as the first form of prevention. Knowing the signs and types will help you determine what your child is going through and what must be done to prevent it. Knowing what they are dealing with will also give you a better idea of how to proceed with teaching them better social and emotional skills and whether school administration must be involved or not.

There are two broad categories of bullying: direct and indirect. Direct bullying occurs face-to-face. The bully acts as the primary handler and oppressor. It can involve physical assault, harassment, and injuries.

An indirect form of bullying involves others too. It mainly consists of the passing of insults or spreading rumors. It inflicts harm to one's social reputation, self-esteem, and relationships.

Types of Bullying

Physical Bullying

Of the many types, physical bullying is the most common form of bullying. In this type, the bully uses physical actions to attain power over the victim. They also use it to hold that power and keep control of their targets. Physical bullies happen to be stronger, bigger, and more aggressive than other types of bullies. They use kicking, hitting, slapping, punching, shoving, and other similar attacks to bully their targets.

Since it all happens in front of many others and the effects are visible in the form of bruises, nosebleeds, and broken bones, physical bullying is the easiest to identify.

There are stronger and more stringent rules in place for this type of bullying. As for the victim, this is the worst form of bullying they can experience and not only affects them mentally but also takes a toll on their health. If the bullying happens frequently, the child may start to bleed internally or suffer from fractures in their hands or feet. This must be stopped at the earliest, and as a parent, you must report it to the authorities right away.

Verbal Bullying

The second type of bullying is verbal bullying. Perpetrators of this type of bullying rely on words, name-calling, and statements to gain power over their victim. They seek control by trying to use insults and slurs. These are meant to belittle, hurt, and demean the victim. Verbal bullies are particular about who they choose to bully. Since they aren't always the largest, they rely on the victim's looks, actions, or behavior. According to them, easy prey is someone that has special needs, has no friends, or is a bit weird around people.

Unlike physical bullying, verbal bullying is difficult to identify as there are no injuries or bruises in plain sight. The bully is often smart enough to get to their victims when few people are around. This makes catching them harder. Bullies use fear to silence their victims and scare them that they would have to face the consequences worse than this if they tried to tell someone. When the bullied try to talk about it with their friends or parents, they are told to simply "ignore" the bully, and eventually, they will stop. But this isn't always the case.

Relational Bullying

Another type of bullying that's prevalent in schools and colleges is relational bullying. This is an indirect form of bullying. During one study, it was found that girls are more involved in this type of bullying as opposed to boys that are more inclined towards hurting their victim physically. Many people know of relational bullying and social bullying. It is centered on trying to achieve a high ground and social standing by diminishing the reputation of others. This is rather petty and can involve the spreading of false rumors both in school and on social media. Since gossip travels fast, many begin to believe that it's too, and therefore, the victim gets mocked, ridiculed, or humiliated.

Social Bullying

Social bullying is also hard to decode as the abuse isn't visible. Even young children that are in elementary school are known to use this form of bullying. They make faces at the child or mimic their actions that make bystanders have a laugh and cause the bullied humiliation. Bullies tell others not to befriend the victim so that they may be excluded from social standing altogether.

Cyberbullying

Cyberbullying happens online. When a tween or teen gets mocked, made fun of, or humiliated on any social media platform, it is classified as cyberbullying. If you are friends with your kid on social media, it will be easier for you to track who comments on your child's status, pictures, and videos or via chat messages. Bullies can use threats and try to harass the target. It could also be an adult, like a high school senior or college-goer. Bullies may also simply stalk their target and keep track of their whereabouts all the time.

Examples of cyberbullying include:
- Making online threats.
- Posting hurtful and embarrassing images and videos.
- Sending scary text messages or emails.

Since kids are always glued to their phones all day long and have this unhealthy habit of posting everything online, cyberbullying is a growing issue. Harassers and bullies can hide behind fake IDs, and therefore, it becomes harder to track.

Nonetheless, there are strict rules against bullying online. Bullies feel empowered when they can hide behind a screen and remain anonymous. Kids from a different race, religion, have weight issues, suffer from disabilities, or have different sexual orientations are more prone to getting bullied online. The consequences of cyberbullying can be damaging.

Sexual Bullying

Sexual bullying involves repeated, humiliating, and harmful actions that target victims sexually. Examples of this type of bullying include name-calling, vulgar gestures, crude comments, uninvited touching, sexual prepositioning, and pornographic material. Bullies can act rudely and pass rude comments about someone's appearance, sexual development, attractiveness, and sexual activity.

Sexual bullying, in extreme cases, opens doors to physical assault. Girls are often the target of sexual bullying by both boys and girls. Boys might take advantage of girls by stalking them, touching them inappropriately, or pass mean comments about their bodies. Girls get called slut, tramp, trash, whore, and other things by fellow girls, and this also continues online.

There is also the danger of sexting that can turn to bully and blackmail. Both guys and girls are known to prey on naïve kids, play with their sentiments via texting, and then try to make advances. Later, they use the same texts to blackmail them and request more favors. Some boys see this as an open opportunity to sexually assault.

Prejudicial Bullying

Finally, there is prejudicial bullying that is more targeted. Here, the bully singles out those from a different race, social standing, religion, or sexual orientation. Often early childhood experiences cause these beliefs to form. Parents are equally to blame if their child shows no acceptance for kids from other ethnicities or cultures. If the parents show bias and preference, the child will normalize it too.

Therefore, you must talk to your child about different races, the effect of racism, the need for tolerance and acceptance, and how to be just with everyone. Kids who are singled out based on the color of their skin, their hair, or their family background suffer from identity complexes all their life. They feel unaccepted, unloved, and undeserving of all good things. It can even lead to hate crimes if not prevented.

Chapter 6:

Bullying Prevention

As parents and educators, we need to build a substantial shift in our mindsets about how important children and their feelings are. Kids thrive when we nurture their humanity, offer them strategies and means to look after themselves well. They thrive when we teach them the right values to help them identify, regulate, and express their feelings. When parents and educators gain awareness of the complex effects of bullying, we can adapt and teach better ways to cope with the dangers and emotional turmoil that it brings along with itself. We need to strongly address the concerns around bullying and lead the way for a better and safer place for our children. After all, young ones count on us.

It has been noted several times that experiencing bullying upfront at school can impact a child's mental, academic, and emotional state. If somehow, we can create a safe and supportive climate for them to excel and learn, we can prevent all forms of bullying from taking place. One of the most talked-about, highly-recommended, and promising approaches are building social and emotional skills (SEL) in children to foster school connectedness, academic achievement, and improved social well-being.

The Collaborative for Academic, Social, and Emotional Learning has developed a framework that involves five core social and emotional skills promoted by parents. These include:

1. Self-awareness: knowing one's feelings, strengths, thoughts, and limitations
2. Self-management: Knowing how to regulate one's emotions and actions when subjected to stress, impulse, and excess motivation.
3. Relationships skills: Knowing how to communicate, be assertive, resolve conflicts, and problem-solve
4. Social awareness: Knowing how to understand and accept different opinions and perspectives, show empathy, and understand norms
5. Responsible decision making: Knowing how to make constructive and responsible choices that affect personal behavior and social interactions.

How Developing Better Emotional and Social Skills Can Help

Social and emotional learning-based approaches are known to deliver solid and cost-effective results. Several meta-analyses suggest that (Durlak et al., 2011). During one study involving hundreds of thousands of K-12 students, SEL practices showed improvement in self-regulation, emotional well-being, classroom relationships, and compassionate behavior with one another (Domitrovich et al., 2017). SEL practices also promote a reduction in stress levels, anxiety, and emotional distress among children. This helps prevent disruptive behaviors like aggression, bullying, conflicts, anger, and hostile attribution bias. At the same time, it improves creativity, leadership, and academic achievement.

Social and emotional skills include the knowledge, skills, and attitudes for youth to be familiar with and control their emotions and behaviors. It fosters the establishment of responsible decision-making, positive relationships, and improved problem-solving skills. Based on this, it becomes a priority to promote these among school-going kids.

According to OECD's research on social-emotional skills surveying ten to fifteen-year-olds, it is estimated that 19 social-emotional skills are developed among kids if they are provided the right guidance by their parents, educators, and peers. These include the following:

1. Achievement Orientation: Setting high standards
2. Self-control: Avoid distractions and improve focus
3. Responsibility: Honor commitments, and be reliable
4. Persistence: Building perseverance

5. Optimism: Setting positive and optimistic expectations
6. Stress-resistance: Modulating anxiety and remaining calm in a difficult situation
7. Self-reflection: Being aware of inner processes and subjective experiences
8. Critical thinking: Ability to evaluate and interpret information
9. Self-efficacy: Belief in oneself to execute and achieve tasks and goals
10. Emotional control: Regulate temper, irritation, and anger in times of frustration
11. Trust: Having good intentions and forgiving those who wronged
12. Empathy: Showing compassion and kindness towards oneself and others
13. Energy: Approaching everyday challenges with excitement and spontaneity
14. Assertiveness: Being confident in voicing concerns, needs, and opinions
15. Cooperation: Being at peace with others and being interconnected
16. Sociability: Approach others, initiate and maintain social-emotional connections
17. Creativity: Generate novel ways to think or do things
18. Curiosity: Intellectual exploration and being in love with learning

19. Tolerance: Openness to different viewpoints and value diversity

How to Talk With My Child About Bullying

Since the overall goal is to help your child stand up against bullies and cope with the emotional turmoil that it comes with, this section is going to be about how you can have that important conversation with them about bullying.

First up, let your child know that no matter what happens, you are always going to believe them. Let them know that the doors of communication are forever open, and they can come to you to discuss anything that bothers them. Show empathy and compassion and tell them that they shouldn't have to be afraid to go to school because you are always going to have their back.

If a child comes with complaints, looks afraid and stressed, lend them an ear. If they want to avoid talking about it, respect their decision. However, whenever you have the chance, let them know that bullying is never acceptable, and if they know someone going through it, you can help them devise ways to counter it. If they have had fights or social confrontations, don't scold them for standing up and being assertive. If they tell you that they tried to stand up for someone at school, applaud their gesture instead of telling them not to make it their business to watch out for everyone at school.

Let Them Know That You Will Take Action if It Is Needed.

Bullying is often tolerated because adults think it is a transient behavior and the hormones are to be blamed. They recall being aggressive when they were young and paying little heed to what's going on. A parent's job is to offer support. It isn't their place to talk their child down or tell them that they need to grow up. Their job is to provide helpful messages and clarify that any form of bullying, whether verbal, physical, or online, will not be tolerated. A parent's job is also to let the child know that it isn't their fault that they are being bullied. They should never think that.

When talking to your child about bullying and the child seems hesitant to talk or open up, engage in role-playing scenarios. If the child is timid and fears standing up, create a few pretend scenarios where you pretend to be the bully, and the child plays the victim. Ask them what they would say to the bully—practice positive responses to help them decide what to say or do if they are bullied again. The goal should be to try and come up with ways that will deescalate a situation. Tell them that they should try to take away power from the bully because that is the one thing they try to snatch from their victim.

Let your child know that although they might be tempted to come back at the bully with a cheeky reply, they shouldn't. They can't control the bully, but there is something that they can control – their reaction. They have to make a choice. They can either inflame the situation or defuse it. If the bully is using some verbal slurs and they can be ignored, do that. It will defuse the situation. If the verbal slurs are rather personal and the bully deserves to be called out on them, go back to the responses you fashioned while role-playing and use them as your defense.

Bullies pick on children that are lonely and isolated. They appear weak because they have no one to stand up for themselves. It makes the bully feel more powerful. Therefore, teach your kids to reach out to those that are alone or play with themselves. Together, you can form a group and avoid being bullied. You don't have to talk to them or invite them to your house. You can just have them sit with you during lunch or walk with you to class to prevent becoming a target.

You can also use TV shows and storybooks to build social skills. Nearly every teen drama stars a bully and how a weak character stands up to them. Watch those shows with your children and later encourage discussing what happened and what could have been done differently. Discuss the characters in-depth, especially that of the bully and the victim, and try to figure out what made them that.

Provide assertive care. Assertive care involves steps that a parent can take when the child continues to get bullied at school despite incorporating the strategies mentioned above. This is the final straw and involves a talk with the administration of the school because the child is unable to handle it themselves, and the bullies don't seem to stop. This is crucial and important because parents that ignore acts of bullying risk breaking the sacred parent-child bond. A child feels like they can't rely on their sole guardians anymore. They feel abandoned by their parents. As a parent, it is your job to advocate for your child. They should be able to rely on you for all their problems. They should know that you will always have their back and will do whatever it takes to get you out of this emotional and mental turmoil.

What Assertive Steps Must You Take?

- Keep a track of the events that took place. Gather as much information as possible about those who were involved in the bullying so that you can appear prepared when you confront the administration. If there are bruises and injuries, take pictures of them and mark them with a date.
- Let the administration or school personnel know of your concerns.
- Connect with the class teacher and see what can be done to prevent instances of bullying. Be cooperative without acting aggressive, hostile, and make it your aim to find out the details of

what happened by chatting with a few close friends or classmates of your child who witnessed the assault.

- Read up about the code of conduct that the school has and what the school's policies on bullying are. See if they are being enforced or not.
    - Do the children know the rules?
    - Do teachers and counselors talk about them in detail during class or not.
- Parents that appear hostile or aggressive seek a confrontation with the bully and their parents. But before doing that assess the degree of openness.
    - Are they willing to discuss the wrongdoings of their child?
    - Are they aware of the fact that their child is a bully?
    - Are they willing to do something about it or not?

Chapter 7:

Empowering Kids to Stand Up for Themselves and Others

As parents, it is hard to imagine a child going through the mental and emotional trauma that comes with bullying. No child deserves to feel like they aren't loved, weak, or unaccepted. They are too young to be introduced to hate, racism, and jealousy. They deserve all the love they can because, sooner or later, the world is going to get to them.

Bullying can have a detrimental effect on the well-being of your child. As discussed previously, we need to set stringent rules to eradicate this evil from all schools and academic institutions. As a parent, your primary instinct has always been to protect your child. You have raised them well so far, but what about when they start to go to school? You can't be with them all the time. Do they know how to take care of themselves when they are alone? Can you rely on them to take a stand for them if they are ever bullied? Do you think they have it in them to call out the bully and report them to an adult? Do you think they will come to your aid and want you to fight their battles?

Of course, as a parent, you will want to confront the bully yourself and put them in their place if the need is but before you go doing that, think about how it is going to affect your child's self-esteem. What will the other kids at school think about them? They will forever be labeled as mama's boy or dad's pet if other kids see them relying on your support to counter bullying.

Besides, you can't be with them when they move out or start college. They will have to learn to stand up for themselves eventually. So why not start early?

In this final chapter of the book, we are going to talk about the many ways you can prepare your child to stand up to a bully. Teach them how they can positively counter and handle bullies alone. Skills such as resilience and assertiveness are going to help them become independent and rely on their sound judgment. This is what we call supportive care. Instead of jumping in, you empower your child to deal with their problems themselves and not be afraid to stand up for themselves and others. School should be a safe place for all. Help your child make it one.

It's Time to Stand Up!

It isn't abnormal that victims of bullying feel sacred to stand up to a bully. Unlike you, they have faced the bullying first hand and know of the power and control the bully has over them and others. They think they aren't strong enough to stand up for themselves and, therefore, pretend that it isn't happening or affecting them. However, the longer they wait to say something, the longer the bullying persists. Remember how we talked about the bully fueling themselves with all the fear and pain they inflict on others? Let your child know that their silence is only going to make the bully stronger.

Therefore, the first thing to do is act fast. If it is the first time they have been bullied, tell them to stand up the next time and not let it happen for the third time. Tell them that retaliation isn't the answer but rather a confident, cool-headed response is. For example, if a bully comes up to them and tries to verbally abuse them, instead of trying to come up with a meaner statement, say something off-the-hook like, "Knock it off," or "That's not funny!" This will disarm the bully and perhaps, even become a mockery in front of others.

Secondly, let your child know that a bully knows when someone feels victimized. A defeated posture, emotional comeback, and weak body language are all signs that indicate that a victim has lost or near the breaking point. Therefore, practice staying calm, strong, and non-emotional. The goal is not to see the victim breaking down. Staying calm and composed will tell the bully that their actions aren't effective.

Maintain steady eye contact and reply to the bully by calling them by their name in a loud but controlled manner. Tell the bully that if they don't stop with their shenanigans, you will tell an adult on them. Most kids will want to avoid doing that but let your child know that it is acceptable behavior, and they shouldn't feel ashamed in doing so.

The next sane thing to do is try to ignore the bully. The reaction is the one thing that the bully expects from you. Don't let them have it. Not reacting or appearing cool when someone says something hurtful is one of the smartest responses to bullying and harassment. Bullies, especially those who are backed by fellow bullies, crave a reaction. They want the victim to cry, scream or pee their pants. They want to make the victim cry so that bystanders know how powerful they can be. If your child offers the response they are after, things will escalate from there, giving the bully more power.

On the other hand, if your child keeps walking their path with their head held high, the bullying will eventually stop, and the bully will start to find another target. They will lose interest in attacking someone that doesn't seem to get affected.

Bullies don't expect your child to stand up to them. Their former experience has assured them that every victim is going to run for their parents. They deliberately target those that appear weaker than them. They know that someone that appears weak is easy to intimidate and manipulate. Conversely, when a victim stands up and tells the bully to stop their abuse upfront, it can startle them a little. If your child appears confident and convinces the bully that they aren't the ones to be preyed upon, they will take a step back. Teach your child to appear strong and tell the bully that they can't walk all over them.

Find allies. Children who have few friends or prefer to stay alone are more prone to bullying. A bully knows that no one will come to their defense if they go after them, making them an easy target. Some stories suggest that if one of the bystanders intervenes and tells the bully that it's their friend, they are more likely to stop. Therefore, tell your child to befriend like-minded people and avoid staying alone during lunch or after school.

Tell your child not to cry as that is the satisfaction the bully is after. They want to see the victim getting upset. If your child can calmly walk away, not retaliate, and engage their attention elsewhere, bullies are less likely to go after them. They target someone that is emotionally weak and alone.

Being funny and laughing right along with a bully shows that you are confident about who you are. Letting the bully see that too tells them that you aren't bothered by what they think or say about you. You have accepted your flaws and don't see them as flaws anymore. When a victim has the confidence to laugh along with the bully, it diffuses the power a bully has over their victim. Encourage your child to do that; however, remind them to only rely on this tactic when they are around other people. A bully doesn't have tolerance for being mocked and might retaliate more harshly. You want your child to have witnessed around so that if they decide to report the abuse, later on, they have solid evidence to produce.

Your child should also know how they can escape the situation. If they feel defenseless and fear that they will be physically assaulted, tell them to look around and see if they can find an exit to escape when the bully is distracted. When the time comes, tell them to make a run for the exit and, if possible, throw things at the bully so that they don't catch up after you and stumble. As soon as you are out of the corner or empty classroom, make a lot of noise and gather a crowd. A bully doesn't want you to attract attention. They want to be the ones to gather crowds.

Tell your child to avoid bullying hotspots. Although you can't be certain, there are some places where incidences of bullying are more prevalent. For example, the back of the bus is a well-known spot. Then there are locker rooms, bathrooms, empty classrooms, vacant hallways, playground corners, etc., that are all known as stakeouts for bullies. Your child must avoid going to these places alone or take a buddy or two along to avoid being bullied.

Conclusion

As children aren't prepared to deal with bullying and harassment early in life, the very first incident can be both shocking and traumatizing. Being bullied isn't fun. It has been known to cause tweens and teenagers to develop mental health issues like stress, anxiety, and depression. It takes away power from them. The victims are left feeling unwanted, isolated, and embarrassed. If not given the proper guidance and the right set of skills, they can never learn to stand up for themselves or others being bullied.

This book looks at the makings of the victim, bully, and bystander. It teaches parents to notice the warning signs and take appropriate steps. Despite being one of the biggest nuisances in schools today, bullying is still prevalent in schools and colleges, and more than half of the students have been a victim of it. Although better laws and practices are in motion today, it still isn't enough to rely on just them.

As parents, you have an important job to do! Teach kids how to fight, prevent, and stand up against bullying. It all begins with building healthy social and emotional skills (SEL). SEL helps students make informed decisions, regulate their emotions better, and deal with incidents of bullying in a healthy and mature way. Learning better social and emotional skills can help them thrive in school as well as their lives later on. As kids aren't born with the knowledge to manage their emotions, these skills can help them problem-solve, be assertive, and stand up against a bully. It can help them navigate positive friendships and relationships with their friends, teachers, and parents.

The more equipped they are, the better their chances of doing their part and nip the evils of bullying in the bud! Thank you for giving this a read. I hope you loved it too because I certainly enjoyed writing it. It would make me the happiest if you would take a moment to leave an honest review. All you have to do is visit the site from where you purchased it. It's that simple! It doesn't have to be a full-fledged paragraph, just a few words will do too. Your few words will help others decide if this is what they should be reading too.

Thank you for giving this a read. I hope you loved it too because I certainly enjoyed writing it. It would make me the happiest if you would take a moment to leave an honest review. All you have to do is visit the site from where you purchased it. It's that simple! It doesn't have to be a full-fledged paragraph, just a few words will do too. Your few words will help others decide if this is what they should be reading too. Thank you in advance and best of luck with your parenting excursions. Surely, every moment is a joyous one with a kid.

References

4 positive lessons for kids on how to stand up to bullying. (n.d.). Www.ourfamilywizard.com. https://www.ourfamilywizard.com/blog/4-positive-lessons-kids-how-stand-bullying

Bullying and the bystander - just say YES - bullying bystanders. (2016, February 19). Just Say YES. https://justsayyes.org/bullying/bullying-and-the-bystander/

Bullying statistics. (2020, November). Www.pacer.org. https://www.pacer.org/bullying/info/stats.asp

Bystanders are essential to bullying prevention and intervention. (2019, September 24). StopBullying.gov; StopBullying.gov. https://www.stopbullying.gov/resources/research-resources/bystanders-are-essential

Divecha, D. (2019, October 29). *What are the best ways to prevent bullying in schools?* Greater Good. https://greatergood.berkeley.edu/article/item/what_are_the_best_ways_to_prevent_bullying_in_schools

Domitrovich, C. E., Durlak, J. A., Staley, K. C., & Weissberg, R. P. (2017). Social-Emotional competence: An essential factor for promoting positive adjustment and reducing risk in school children. Child Development, 88(2), 408–416. https://doi.org/10.1111/cdev.12739

Dryden-Edwards, R. (2008). *Bullying facts, statistics, prevention & effects.* MedicineNet. https://www.medicinenet.com/bullying/article.htm

DuBois-Maahs, J. (2018, November 21). *Types of bullying and its effects | talkspace.* Talkspace. https://www.talkspace.com/blog/types-of-bullying-effects-solutions/

Durlak, J. A., Weissberg, R. P., Dymnicki, A. B., Taylor, R. D., & Schellinger, K. B. (2011). The impact of enhancing students' social and emotional learning: A meta-analysis of school-based universal interventions. Child Development, 82(1), 405–432. https://doi.org/10.1111/j.1467-8624.2010.01564.x

Facts about bullying. (2019, September 24). StopBullying.gov; StopBullying.gov. https://www.stopbullying.gov/resources/facts

Fraser-Thrill, R. (2020, September 15). *Some children are more likely to be victimized than others.* Verywell Family. https://www.verywellfamily.com/characteristic

s-of-a-typical-victim-of-bullying-3288501#citation-4

Gini, G., & Pozzoli, T. (2013). *Bullied children and psychosomatic problems: A meta-analysis.* PEDIATRICS, 132(4), 720–729. https://doi.org/10.1542/peds.2013-0614

Gordon, S. (2017, October 27). *6 types of bullying every parent should know about.* Verywell Family; Verywellfamily. https://www.verywellfamily.com/types-of-bullying-parents-should-know-about-4153882

Gordon, S. (2019, August 17). *Why kids who witness bullying often do not report it.* Verywell Family. https://www.verywellfamily.com/reasons-why-bystanders-remain-silent-460741

Gordon, S. (2020, December 18). *Is hazing really a form of bullying?* Verywell Family. https://www.verywellfamily.com/bullying-and-hazing-is-there-a-difference-460505

Gordon, S. (2021, February 18). *Teach your child how to deal with a bully.* Verywell Family. https://www.verywellfamily.com/plan-for-standing-up-to-bullying-460810

Hong, J. S., Espelage, D. L., Grogan-Kaylor, A., & Allen-Meares, P. (2011). *Identifying potential mediators and moderators of the association between child maltreatment and bullying perpetration and victimization in school*. Educational Psychology Review, 24(2), 167–186. https://doi.org/10.1007/s10648-011-9185-4

How to talk to your children about bullying. (n.d.). Www.unicef.org. https://www.unicef.org/end-violence/how-talk-your-children-about-bullying

Kungu, E. (n.d.). *Difference between teasing and bullying | difference between*. Difference Between. http://www.differencebetween.net/language/difference-between-teasing-and-bullying/

Lee, A. M. I. (2019, August 5). *The difference between teasing and bullying*. Understood.org; Understood. https://www.understood.org/en/friends-feelings/common-challenges/bullying/difference-between-teasing-and-bullying

Lewis, R. (2021, January 22). *Recognizing the types of bullying and potential effects*. Healthline. https://www.healthline.com/health/childrens-health/types-of-bullying

Loveless, B. (2010). *Bullying epidemic: Facts, statistics and prevention*. Educationcorner.com. https://www.educationcorner.com/bullying-facts-statistics-and-prevention.html

Mangel, L. (2018, February 23). *10 ways to empower kids to stand up to bullying*. Bosco-App. https://www.boscoapp.com/single-post/2018/02/23/10-Ways-To-Empower-Kids-To-Stand-Up-To-Bullying

Polanin, J. R., Espelage, D. L., & Pigott, T. D. (2012). *A meta-analysis of school-based bullying prevention programs' effects on bystander intervention behavior.* School Psychology Review, 41(1), 47–65. https://doi.org/10.1080/02796015.2012.12087 375

Rowley, E., Chandler, S., Baird, G., Simonoff, E., Pickles, A., Loucas, T., & Charman, T. (2012). *The experience of friendship, victimization and bullying in children with an autism spectrum disorder: Associations with child characteristics and school placement.* Research in Autism Spectrum Disorders, 6(3), 1126–1134. https://doi.org/10.1016/j.rasd.2012.03.004

Social emotional learning helps prevent bullying. (2020, March 26). StopBullying.gov. https://www.stopbullying.gov/blog/2020/03/25/social-emotional-learning-helps-prevent-bullying

Study shows bullying affects both bystanders and target | penn state university. (2011). Psu.edu. https://news.psu.edu/story/154651/2011/10/11/study-shows-bullying-affects-both-bystanders-and-target

The difference between teasing and bullying | prevnet - canada's authority on bullying. (2019). Prevnet.ca.

https://www.prevnet.ca/bullying/educators/th e-difference-between-teasing-and-bullying

Understanding bullying: The victim. (n.d.). UniversalClass.com. Retrieved May 10, 2021, from https://www.universalclass.com/articles/psych ology/understanding-bullying-the-victim.htm

What is the difference between bullying and harassment? (n.d.). Www.pacer.org. https://www.pacer.org/bullying/info/question s-answered/bullying-harassment.asp

What you need to know about bullying. (n.d.). The Center for Parenting Education. Retrieved May 10, 2021, from https://centerforparentingeducation.org/library -of-articles/handling-bullying-issues/what-you-need-to-know-about-bullying/

Whitson, S. (2013, November 19). 6 reasons why bystanders choose not to intervene to stop bullying. HuffPost; HuffPost. https://www.huffpost.com/entry/six-reasons-why-bystander_b_4295181

Youth risk behavior surveillance system (YRBSS). (2020, October). Centers for Disease Control and Prevention. https://www.cdc.gov/healthyyouth/data/yrbs/ index.htm

Made in the USA
Las Vegas, NV
29 April 2022

48155514R00044